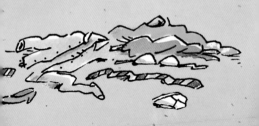

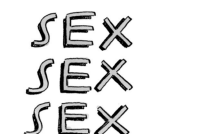

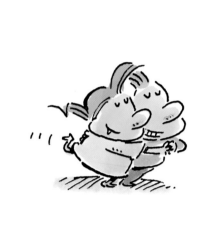

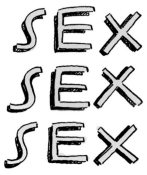

Ariel Books

♥

Andrews and McMeel

Kansas City

Frontispiece by Joe Stites

ISBN:0-8362-3116-3

Library of Congress Catalog Card Number: 94-72874

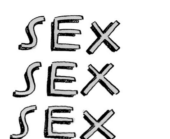

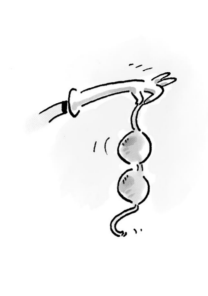

Anything worth doing well is
worth doing slowly.
—*Gypsy Rose Lee*

The tragedy is when you've got sex
in the head instead of down where
it belongs.
—*D. H. Lawrence*

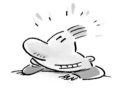

Shared laughter is erotic too.
—*Marge Piercy*

The spirit is often most free when the body is satiated with pleasure; indeed, sometimes the stars shine more brightly seen from the gutter than from the hilltop.
—*W. Somerset Maugham*

Sexuality is the lyricism of the masses.
—*Charles Baudelaire*

I thought *coq au vin* was love in a lorry.
—*Victoria Wood*

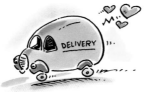

I'm at the age where food has taken the place of sex in my life. In fact, I've just had a mirror put over my kitchen table.
—*Rodney Dangerfield*

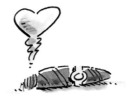

From the moment I was six I felt
sexy. And let me tell you it was
hell, sheer hell, waiting to do
something about it.
　　—*Bette Davis*


Sometimes a cigar is just a cigar.
　　—*Sigmund Freud*

I used to be Snow White—but I drifted.
—*Mae West*


And the lovers lie abed with all their griefs in their arms.
—*Dylan Thomas*

A kiss can be a comma, a question mark, or an exclamation point. That's basic spelling that every woman ought to know.
—*Mistinguett*

I'm suggesting we call sex something else, and it should include everything from kissing to sitting close together.
—*Shere Hite*

Sex is an emotion in motion.
—*Mae West*

Amoebas at the start
Were not complex
They tore themselves apart
And started Sex.
—*Arthur Guiterman*

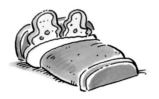

The right diet directs sexual energy into the parts that matter.
—*Barbara Cartland*

Give me chastity and continence, but not just now.
—*St. Augustine*

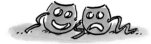

The reason so many women fake orgasms is that so many men fake foreplay.
      —*Graffiti*


If I have to cry, I think of my sex life. If I have to laugh, I think of my sex life.
      —*Glenda Jackson*

Scratch a lover, and find a foe.
 —*Dorothy Parker*


Graze on my lips; and if those hills
 be dry,
Stray lower, where the pleasant
 fountains lie.
 —*William Shakespeare*

The last important human activity
not subject to taxation.
—*Russell Baker*

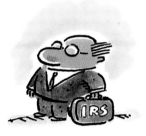

When turkeys mate they think of swans.
—*Johnny Carson*

The difference between pornography and erotica is lighting.
—*Gloria Leonard*

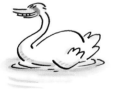

Sex is the great amateur art. The professional, male or female, is frowned on; he or she misses the whole point and spoils the show.
—*David Cort*

The only people who make love all the time are liars.
—*Telly Savalas*

Think of me as a sex symbol for
the men who don't give a damn.
    —*Phyllis Diller*


Make love to every woman you
meet. If you get five per cent on
your outlays, it's a good invest-
ment.
    —*Arnold Bennett*

Of course I flaunt my assets. They are big, but I've always had 'em, pushed 'em up, whacked 'em around. Why not make fun when I've earned a fortune with 'em?
—*Dolly Parton*

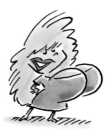

There is nothing like desire for preventing the thing one says from bearing any resemblance to what one has in mind.
—*Marcel Proust*

Nothing is either all masculine or all feminine except having sex.
—*Marlo Thomas*

Sex is good, but not as good as fresh sweet corn.
—*Garrison Keillor*

He was one of those men who come in a door and make any woman with them look guilty.
—*F. Scott Fitzgerald*

It's been so long since I made love,
I can't even remember who gets
tied up.
    —*Joan Rivers*


To succeed with the opposite sex,
tell her you're impotent. She can't
wait to disprove it.
    —*Cary Grant*

As to sex, the original pleasure, I cannot recommend too highly the advantages of androgyny.
—*Jan Morris*

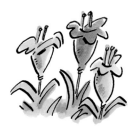

Blondes have the hottest kisses.
Redheads are fair-to-middling
torrid, and brunettes are the
frigidest of all. It's something to
do with hormones, no doubt.
—*Ronald Reagan*

Sexual intercourse began
In nineteen sixty-three
(Which was rather late for me)—
Between the end of the *Chatterley*
  ban
And the Beatles' first LP.
    —*Philip Larkin*

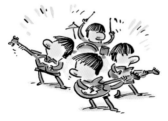

Woe to the man who tries to be
frank in love-making.
   —*George Sand (Amandine-*
      *Aurore-Lucile Dupin)*

Lie back and think of England.
   —*Anonymous (Victorian advice*
      *to women)*

So we think of Marilyn who was every man's love affair with America. Marilyn Monroe who was blonde and beautiful and had a sweet little rinky-dink of a voice and all the cleanliness of all the clean American backyards. She was our angel, the sweet angel of sex, and the sugar of sex came up from her like a resonance of sound in the clearest grain of a violin.

—*Norman Mailer*

I was asked if my first sexual experience was homosexual or heterosexual. I said I was too polite to ask.
　　　—*Gore Vidal*

The poor man's polo.
　　　—*Clifford Odets*

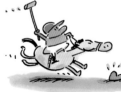

A satisfying sex life is the single most effective protection against heart attacks.
—*Dr. Eugene Scheimann*

It's not the men in my life, it's the life in my men.
—*Mae West*

A clever imitation of love. It has all the action but none of the plot.
—*William Rotsler*

Sex is hardly ever just about sex.
—*Shirley MacLaine*

I wasn't kissing her, I was whispering in her mouth.
—*Chico Marx*

We must act out passion before we can feel it.
—*Jean-Paul Sartre*

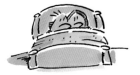

In a society where people get more or less what they want sexually, it is much more difficult to motivate them in an industrialized context, to make them buy refrigerators and cars.

—*William S. Burroughs*

Oh, what lies there are in kisses.
—*Heinrich Heine*

Love is not the dying moan of a
distant violin—it's the triumphant
twang of a bedspring.
—*S. J. Perelman*

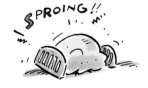

Kissing don't last; cookery do!
  —*George Meredith*


Sex is work.
  —*Andy Warhol*

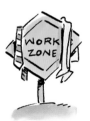

In the case of some women, orgasms take quite a bit of time. Before signing on with such a partner, make sure you are willing to lay aside, say, the month of June, with sandwiches having to be brought in.

—*Bruce Jay Friedman*

The ability to make love frivolously
is the chief characteristic which
distinguishes human beings from
the beasts.
—*Heywood Broun*

I've only slept with men I've been
married to. How many women can
make that claim?
—*Elizabeth Taylor*

Take a perfect circle, caress it and you'll have a vicious circle.

—*Eugène Ionesco*

The perfect lover is one who turns into a pizza at 4:00 A.M.

—*Charles Pierce*

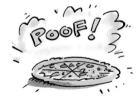

Man survives earthquakes, epidemics, the horrors of disease, and all the agonies of the soul, but for all time his tormenting tragedy is, and will be, the tragedy of the bedroom.

—Leo Tolstoy

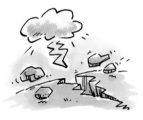

There is no middle-class sexual style for men. What would it be based on? Golfing? Discussing stock options? Attending church? Downing highballs?
    —Edmund White

Nothing risqué, nothing gained.
—*Alexander Woollcott*


If you aren't going all the way, why go at all?
—*Joe Namath*

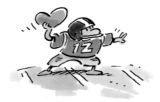

Sex is not only a divine and beautiful activity: it's a murderous activity. People kill each other in bed. Some of the greatest crimes ever committed were committed in bed. And no weapons were used.
—*Norman Mailer*

Is it not strange that desire
should so many years outlive
performance?
        —*William Shakespeare*


Those who restrain desire, do so
because theirs is weak enough to
be restrained.
        —*William Blake*

Ah, if I'd had breasts I could have ruled the world!
—*Julie Harris*


It is certainly very hard to write about sex in English without making it unattractive.
—*Edmund Wilson*

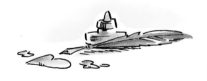

Nature abhors a virgin—a frozen asset.
—*Clare Boothe Luce*

There is no unhappier creature on earth than a fetishist who yearns for a woman's shoe and has to embrace the whole woman.
—*Karl Kraus*

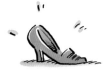

I believe a little incompatibility is the spice of life, particularly if he has income and she is pattable.
—*Ogden Nash*

The prettiest dresses are worn to be taken off.
—*Jean Cocteau*

Personally I know nothing about sex because I've always been married.

—*Zsa Zsa Gabor*

My own belief is that there is hardly anyone whose sexual life, if it were broadcast, would not fill the world at large with surprise and horror.

—*W. Somerset Maugham*

If it weren't for pickpockets, I'd have no sex life at all.
—*Rodney Dangerfield*

You sleep with a guy once and before you know it he wants to take you to dinner.
—*Myers Yori*

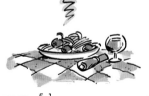

The true feeling of sex is that of
a deep intimacy, but above all of a
deep complicity.
—*James Dickey*


The worst sin—perhaps the only
sin—passion can commit, is to be
joyless.
—*Dorothy L. Sayers*

Everybody lies about sex.
    —*Robert Heinlein*

The great discovery of the age is
that women like it too.
    —*Hugh MacDiarmid*

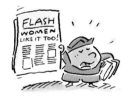

Sleeping alone, except under doctor's orders, does much harm. Children will tell you how lonely it is sleeping alone. If possible you should always sleep with someone you love. You recharge your mutual batteries free of charge.

—*Marlene Dietrich*

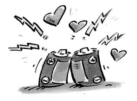

In my sex fantasy, nobody ever loves me for my mind.
　　—*Nora Ephron*

Chastity is curable, if detected early.
　　—*Anonymous*

All really great lovers are articulate,
and verbal seduction is the surest
road to actual seduction.
    —*Marya Mannes*


France is the only place where you
can make love in the afternoon
without people hammering on
your door.
    —*Barbara Cartland*

If you wish,
I shall grow irreproachably tender:
Not a man, but a cloud in trousers!
—*Vladimir Mayakovski*

Great food is like great sex—the
more you have the more you want.
—*Gail Greene*

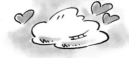

Why do they put the Gideon Bibles only in the bedrooms, where it's usually too late, and not in the barroom downstairs?
— *Christopher Morley*

It is not enough to conquer; one must know how to seduce.
— *Voltaire*

I'm saving the bass player for
Omaha.

—Janis Joplin

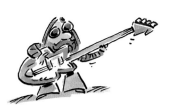

Women complain about sex more often than men. Their gripes fall into two major categories: (1) Not enough (2) Too much.
—*Ann Landers*

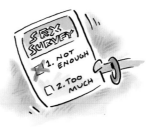

Those people who think good sex is more important to a marriage than good manners will find they are wrong. It is an irony, appreciated only by the French, that good manners are the basis of very good sex. In bed, the two most erotic words in any language are *thank you* and *please*.

—Hubert Downs

Dancing is the perpendicular expression of a horizontal desire.
   —*Anonymous*

I finally had an orgasm . . . and my doctor told me it was the wrong kind.
   —*Woody Allen*

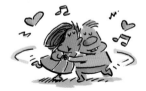

Never underestimate the power of passion.
—*Eve Sawyer*


I wanted to give a woman comfortable clothes that would flow with her body. A woman is closest to being naked when she is well dressed.
—*Coco Chanel*

To err is human—but it feels
divine.
            —*Mae West*


The best cure for hypochondria is
to forget about your own body and
get interested in someone else's.
            —*Goodman Ace*

My dear, it doesn't matter what
they do, so long as they don't do
it in the street and frighten the
horses.
—*Mrs. Patrick Campbell*


I like a man what takes his time.
—*Mae West*

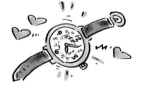

You mustn't force sex to do the work of love or love to do the work of sex.
—*Mary McCarthy*

Marriage has many pains, but celibacy has no pleasures.
—*Samuel Johnson*

The sexual embrace can only be compared with music and with prayer.
—*Havelock Ellis*

In diving to the bottom of pleasure we bring up more gravel than pearls.
—*Honoré de Balzac*

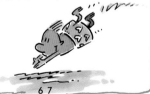

Do not exploit. Do not be exploited. Remember that sex is not out there, but in here, in the deepest layer of your own being. There is not only a morning after—there are also lots of days and years afterward.

—*Jacob Neusner*

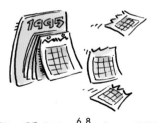

There will be sex after death; we just won't be able to feel it.
—*Lily Tomlin*

Sex ought to be a wholly satisfying link between two affectionate people from which they emerge unanxious, rewarded, and ready for more.
—*Alex Comfort*

The 1950s were ten years of foreplay.

—*Germaine Greer*

Those hot pants of hers were so damned tight, I could hardly breathe.

—*Benny Hill*

Being bald is an unfailing sex
magnet.
—*Telly Savalas*

It's hard for me to get used to
these changing times. I can
remember when the air was clean
and the sex was dirty.
—*George Burns*

Lord, I wonder what fool it was
that first invented kissing!
—*Jonathan Swift*


Thunder and lightning, wars,
fires, plagues, have not done that
mischief to mankind as this
burning lust.
—*Robert Burton*

Be a good animal, true to your
animal instincts.
    —*D. H. Lawrence*


Whoever named it necking was a
poor judge of anatomy.
    —*Groucho Marx*

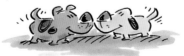

I don't see much of Alfred any
more since he got so interested in
sex.
—*Mrs. Alfred Kinsey*

You sofa-crevice fondler!
—*Peter De Vries*

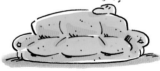

Men make love more intensely
at twenty, but make love better,
however, at thirty.
—*Catherine II of Russia*

Whatever else can be said about
sex, it cannot be called a dignified
performance.
—*Helen Lawrenson*

I tend to believe that cricket is the greatest thing God ever created on earth . . . certainly greater than sex, although sex isn't too bad either.
—*Harold Pinter*

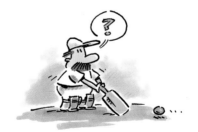

I want to tell you a terrific story about oral contraception. I asked this girl to sleep with me and she said "no."
    —Woody Allen

If it is not erotic, it is not interesting.
    —Fernando Arrabal

Some things are better than sex,
and some are worse, but there's
nothing exactly like it.
  —W. C. Fields


What is beyond Desire, but
Desire?
  —*Gretel Ehrlich*

At certain times I like sex—like
after a cigarette.
      —*Rodney Dangerfield*

Bed is the poor man's opera.
      —*Italian proverb*

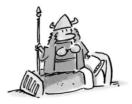

The text of this book was set in Electra
by Snap-Haus Graphics, Dumont,
New Jersey.

Book design by
Diane Stevenson / Snap-Haus Graphics

Illustrations by Joe Stites

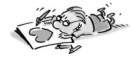